Sam Feels Better Now!

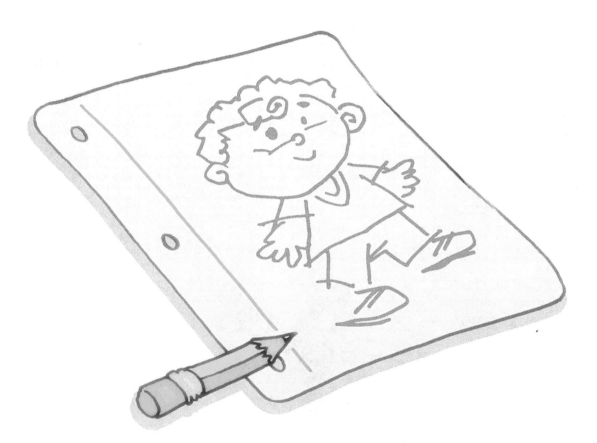

Written by Jill Osborne
Illustrated by Kevin Collier

Sam Feels Better Now! : An Interactive Story for Children
Text copyright (c) 2008 by Jill Osborne.
Illustrations copyright (c) 2008 by Kevin Collier.
All Rights Reserved.
First Printing: July 2008

Library of Congress Cataloging-in-Publication Data

Osborne, Jill, 1978-
  Sam feels better now! : an interactive story for children / by Jill Osborne ; illustrations by Kevin Scott Collier.
    p. cm.
  ISBN-13: 978-1-932690-60-6 (trade paper : alk. paper)
  ISBN-10: 1-932690-60-3 (trade paper : alk. paper)
  1. Psychic trauma in children--Treatment--Juvenile literature. I. Collier, Kevin Scott, ill. II. Title.
  RJ506.P66O64 2008
  618.92'8521--dc22

                        2008012386

Loving Healing Press
5145 Pontiac Trail
Ann Arbor, MI 48105
www.LHPress.com

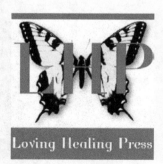

Dedication

This book is dedicated to Inge and Judy who introduced me to play therapy, and to my professors at Georgia State University for all your support. Special Thanks to Kevin Collier and Margot Finke who helped make this book possible.

Introduction

This book presents stage one of trauma therapy for children (Brack 2007). It will help those with psychological injury from abuse or other causes. The intention is for the child to use it in conjunction with a therapist. This can occur over a period of time, not necessarily within one session. Further work may be needed following completion of this book. The therapist is encouraged to follow this program while consulting with caregivers to create a safe, supportive environment for their child and family.

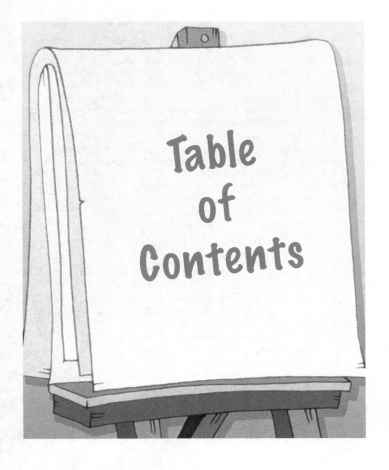

Table of Contents

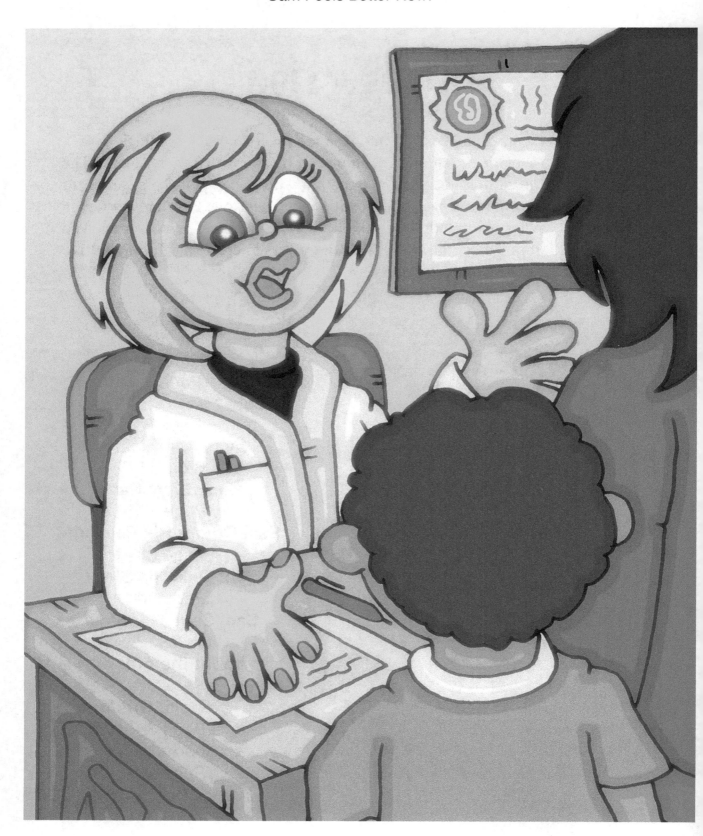

Mrs. Carol is a special therapist who helps kids feel better. One day, when Ms. Carol was in her office, Sam and his mom came to visit her. Ms. Carol smiled at Sam. "How can I help you?" She asked.

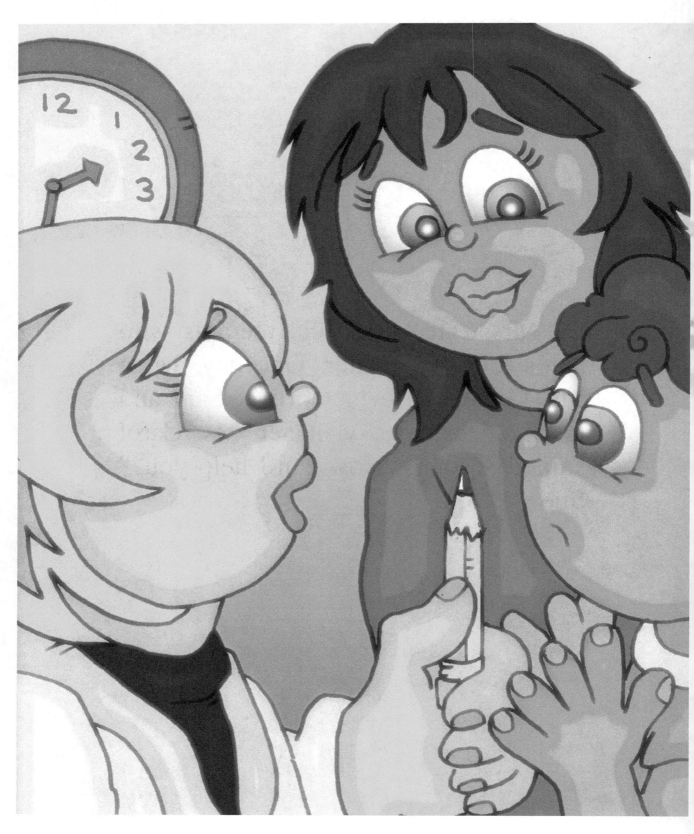

"Sam was scared by something awful," said his mom. "And he's having trouble sleeping. He isn't eating enough either, and he's fighting with some of his friends."

Ms. Carol nodded. "Sam, can you draw me a picture of someone who is scared?"

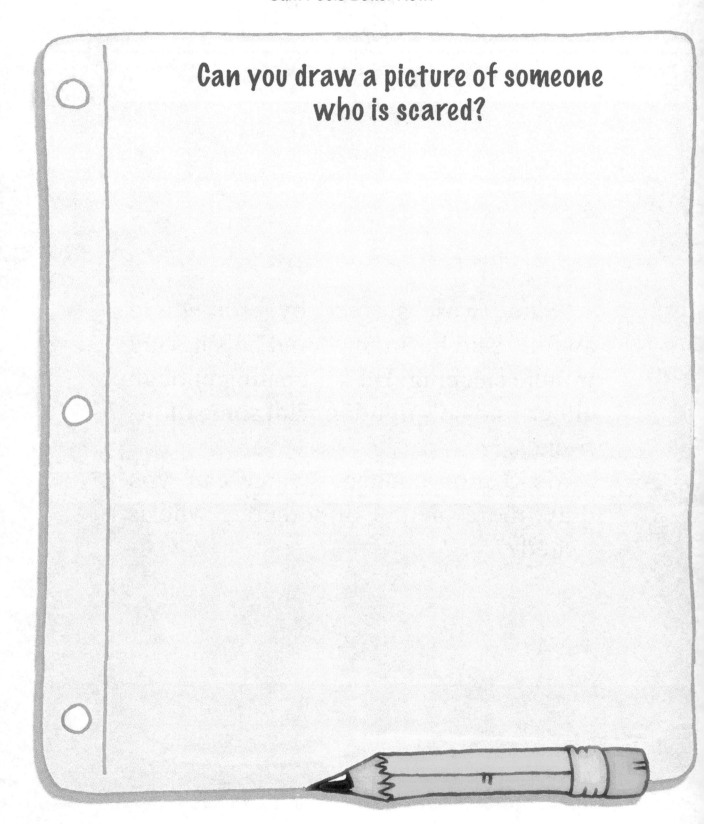

Can you draw a picture of someone who is scared?

When Ms. Carol saw Sam's drawing, she patted his shoulder gently.

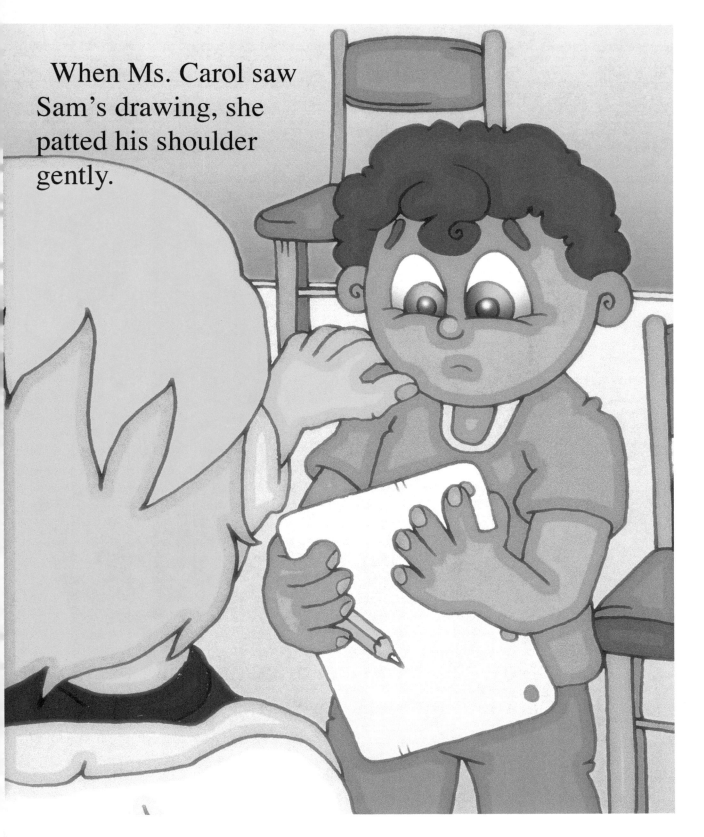

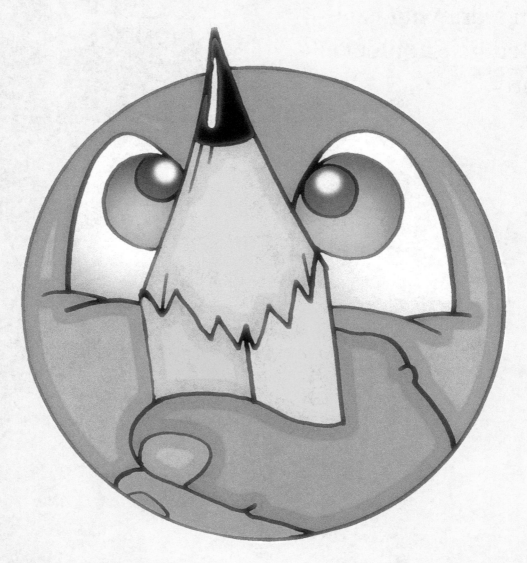

"Now see if you can draw me a picture of something awful or scary."

Can you draw a picture of something awful or scary?

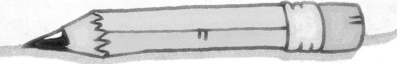

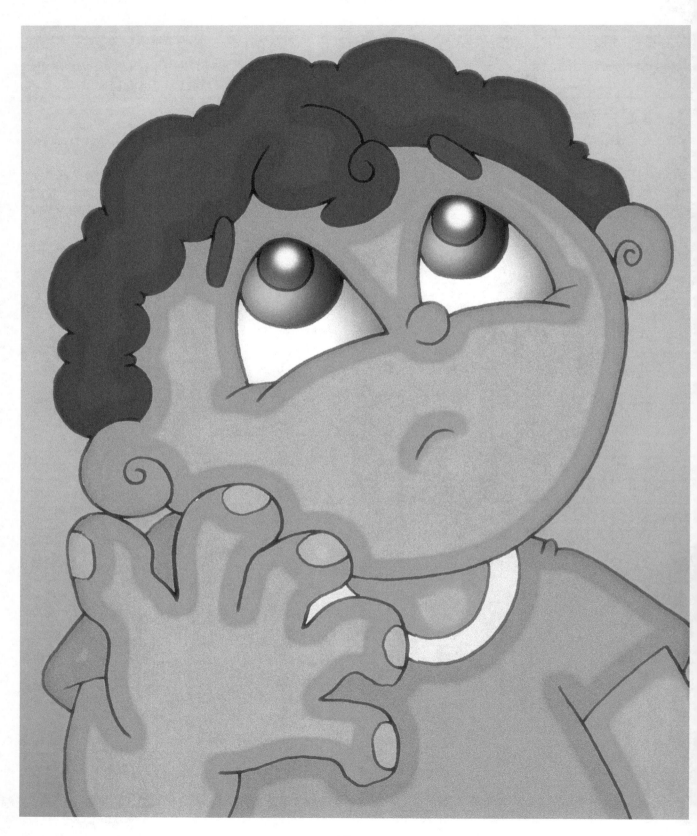

"Why do I feel scared all the time, and can't sleep," Sam asked Ms. Carol," is it normal to feel like this?

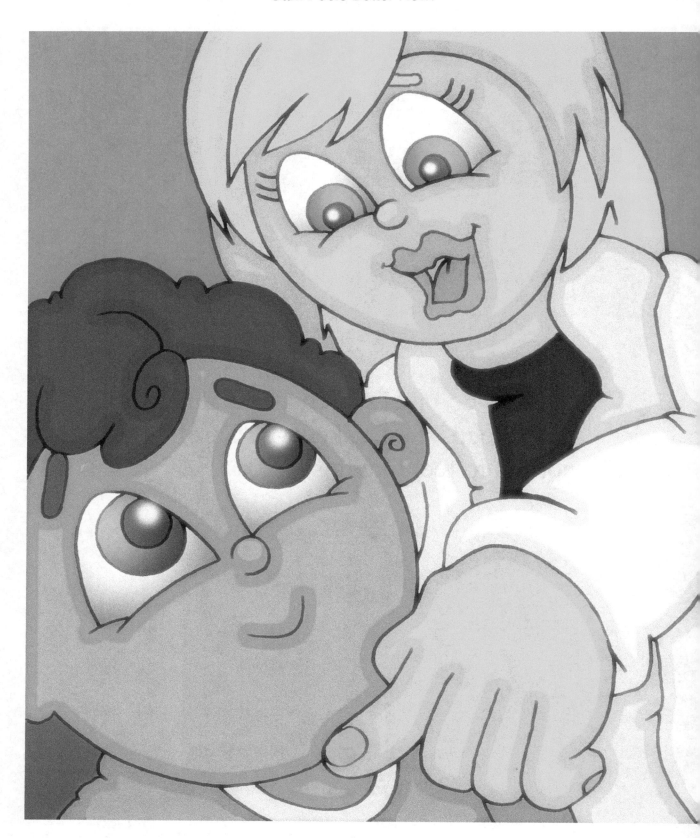

Ms. Carol smiled and reassured him. "Sometimes, when people see something awful, they feel worried and scared, just like you. It's the way some people react to seeing awful things. But there are many things you can do to help you feel better."

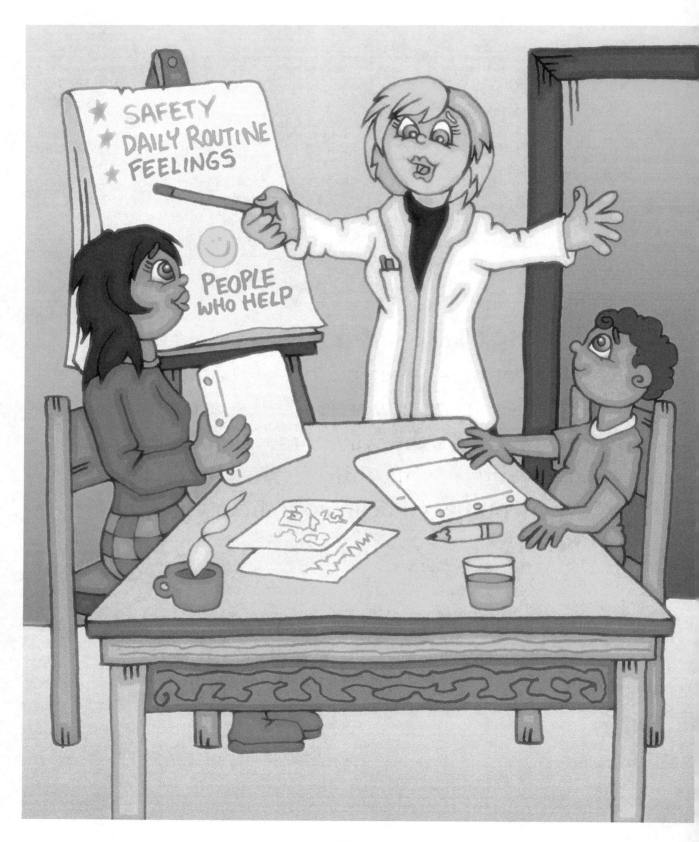

So Ms. Carol began helping Sam learn how to feel better after seeing such an awful event. She began showing him and his mom about safety, a daily routine, feelings, people who can help, ways to relax, and how to tell stories about the things that were bothering him.

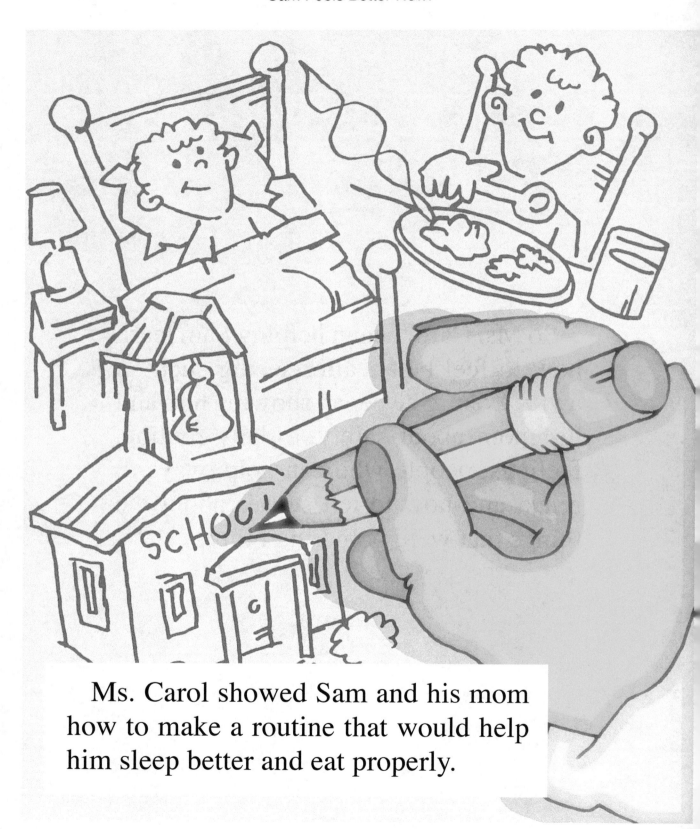

Ms. Carol showed Sam and his mom how to make a routine that would help him sleep better and eat properly.

Ms. Carol talked to Sam and his mom about people who can help Sam if he starts to feel afraid. Sam named friends, family, teachers, and others that can help him.

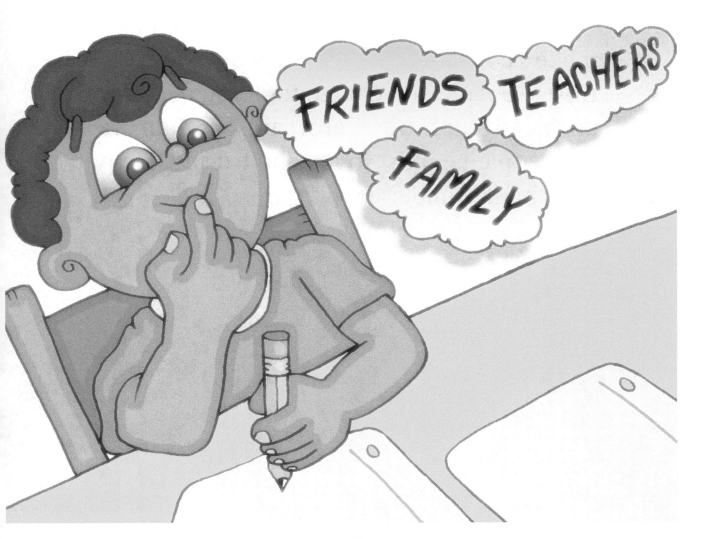

"Sam, I'd like you to draw a picture, or make a collage of the special people you really trust—people you can go to if you feel afraid and need help," Ms. Carol said. So, Sam drew the people he most loved and trusted. He put their names under each figure.

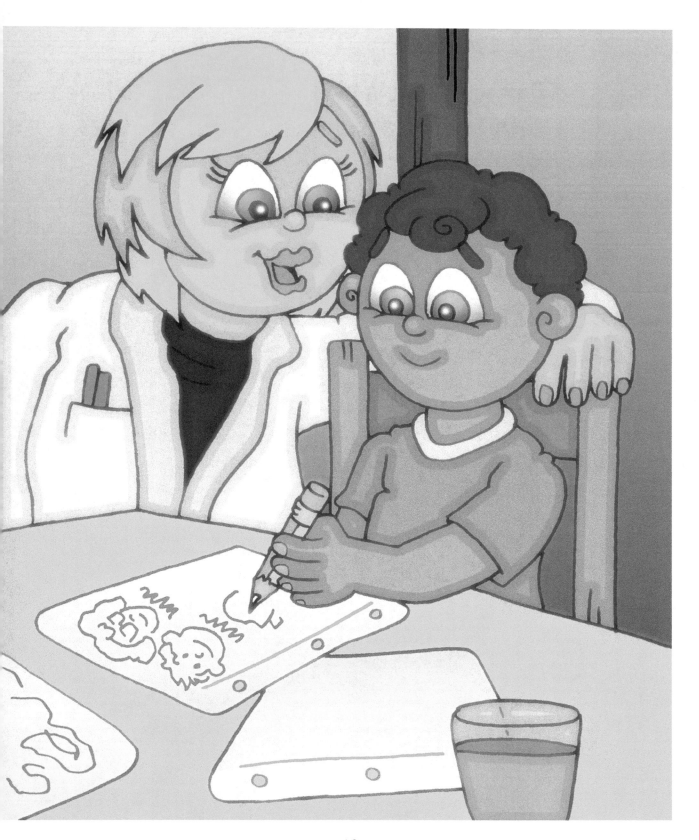

Can you draw a picture or make a collage of people that Sam can love and trust?

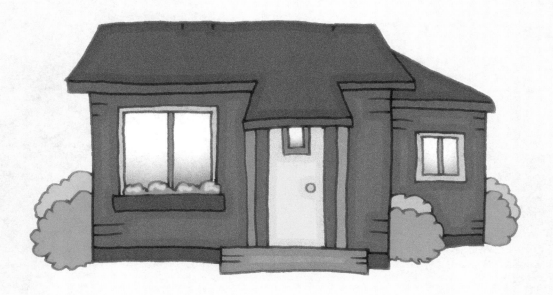

Ms. Carol helped Sam think of ways to stay safe when he is scared. "Where can you go in your house if you want to feel safe?" Ms. Carol asked. Sam drew a picture for her.

Can you draw a picture of a place where Sam can go in his house to feel safe?

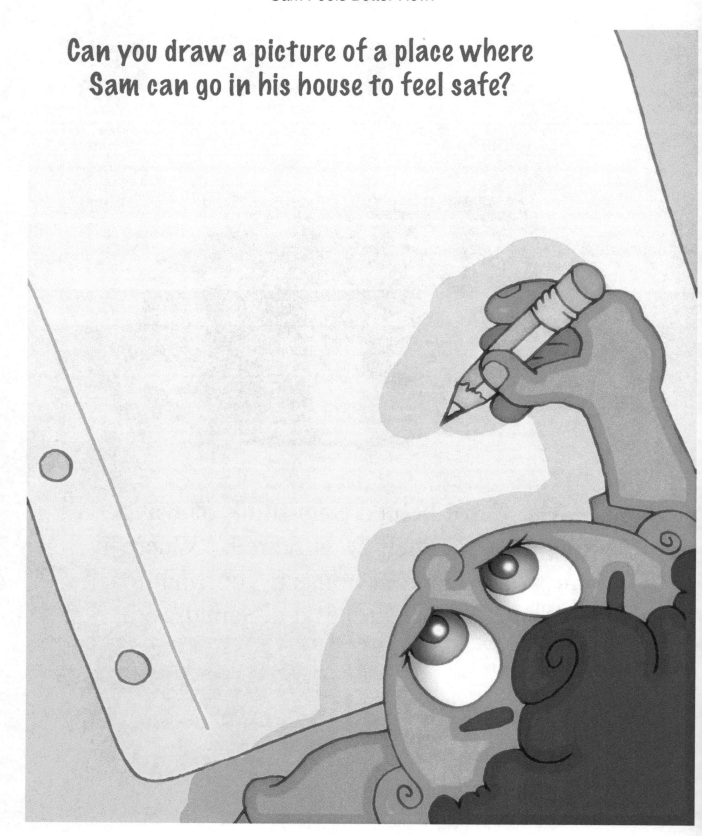

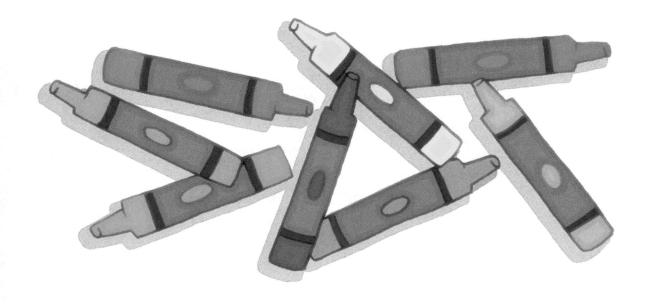

After that, Ms. Carol taught him to understand the feelings he kept having. Sam colored his feelings in circles, like the ones on the next page.

Can you help Sam color his feelings?

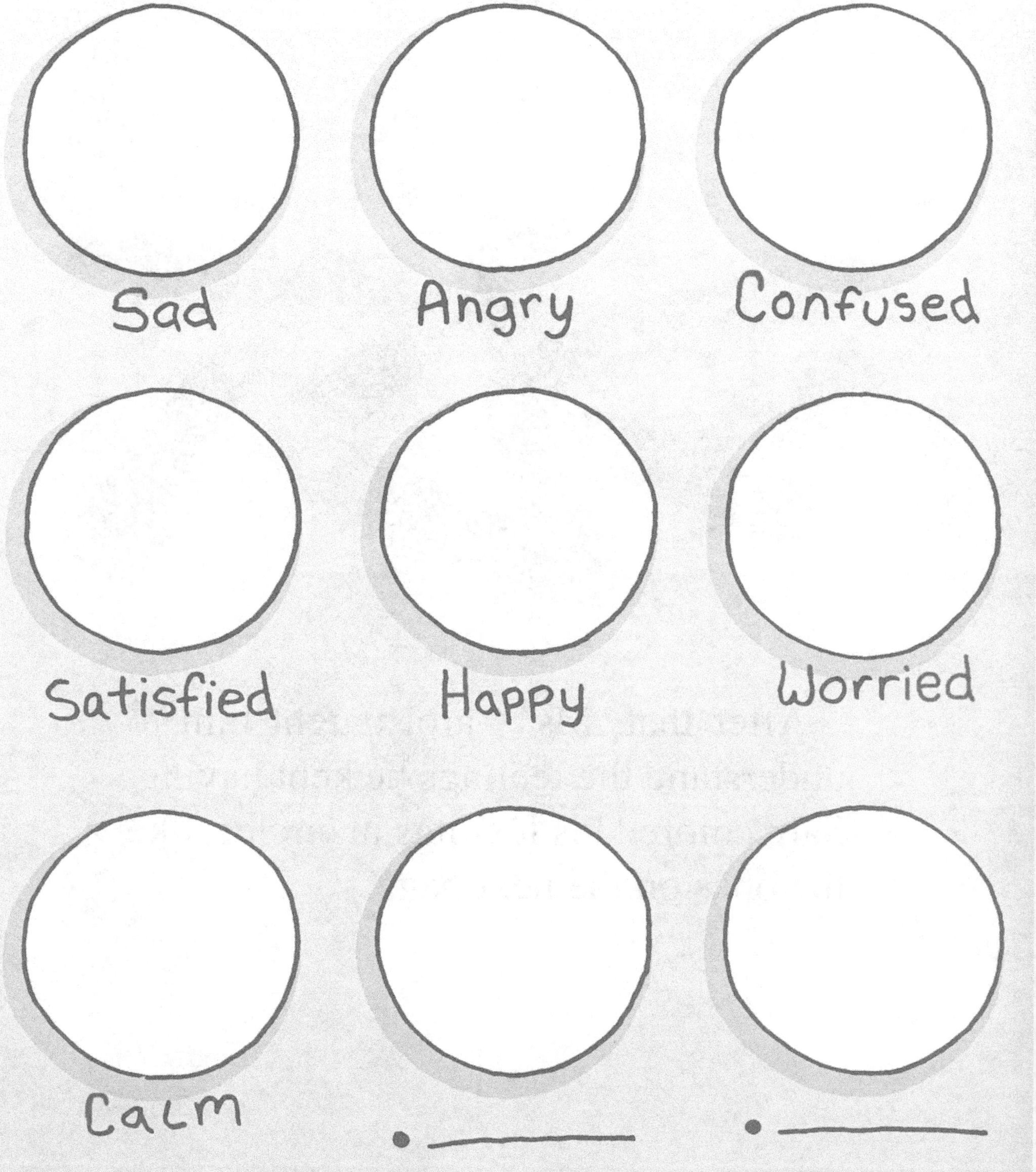

Sad

Angry

Confused

Satisfied

Happy

Worried

Calm

• _____

• _____

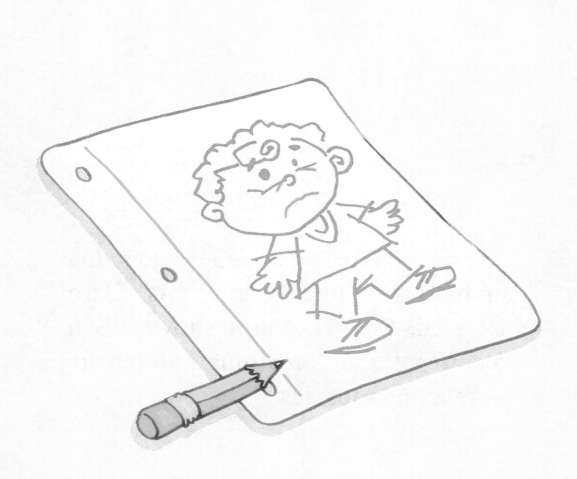

During their session, Sam said, "Sometimes I feel nervous and worried"

"I will show you some ways that can help you feel better," Ms. Carol answered. So Ms. Carol showed Sam ways to relax by breathing and tensing and relaxing muscles.

Can you help Sam by drawing ways that will help him to relax?

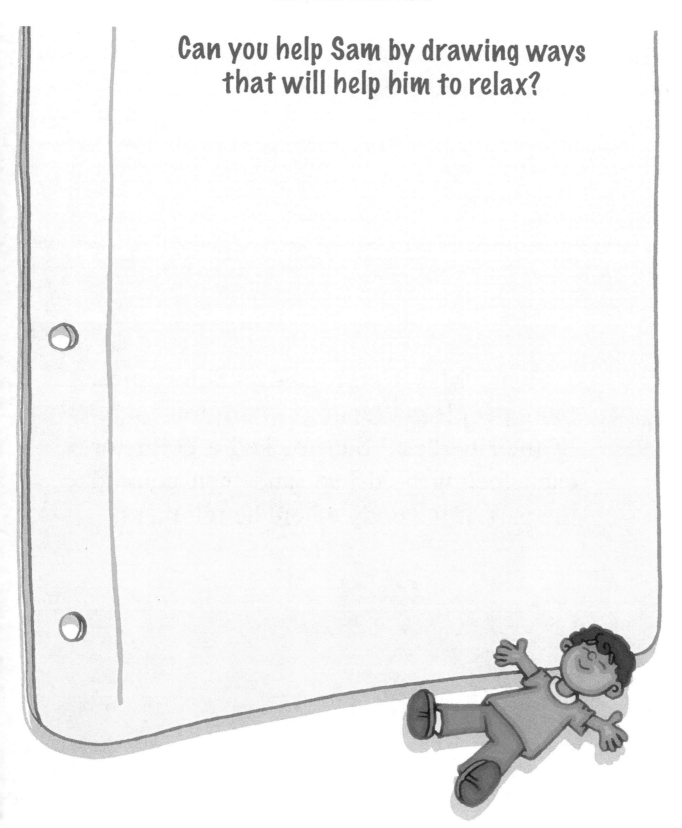

Then, Ms. Carol said, "Sometimes, Sam, people get feelings in different parts of their bodies." Sam picked a color for each feeling he'd had, and then colored the part of the body where he felt them.

Can you help Sam by showing him where to color feelings in his body?

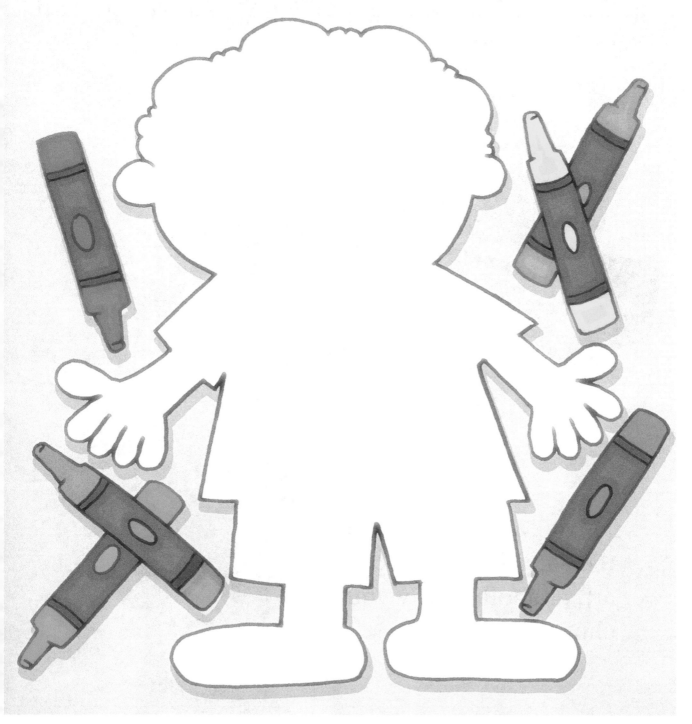

Next, Ms. Carol asked Sam to tell a story about the awful thing that scared him. Choose a way to help Sam tell his story.

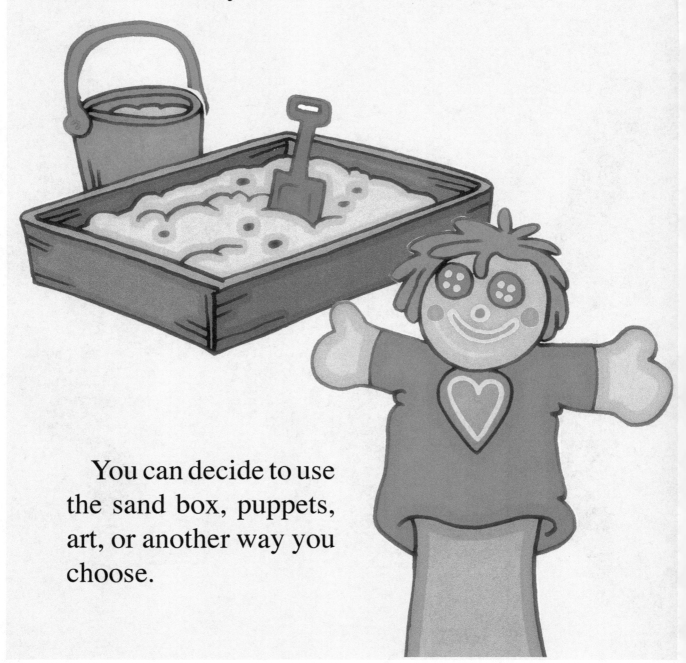

You can decide to use the sand box, puppets, art, or another way you choose.

Can you tell a story about an awful, scary thing that happened? Draw a picture here, or choose another way to tell the story.

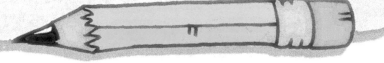

After that, Ms. Carol asked Sam how he felt after telling his story and learning ways to feel better.

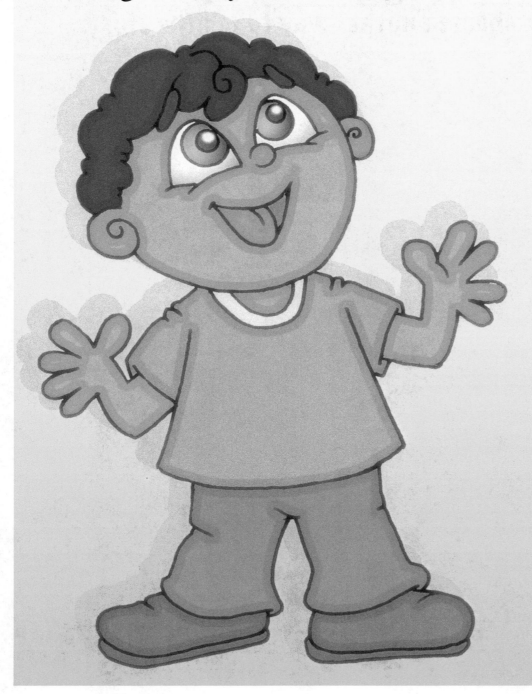

"I feel better now, safer and more relaxed. Better about myself too. I even slept better last night." He grinned.

After that, Ms. Carol met with Sam and his mom once a week.

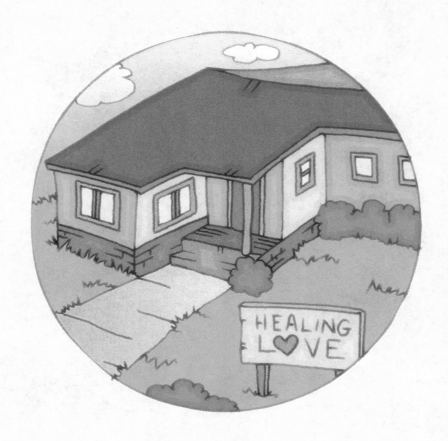

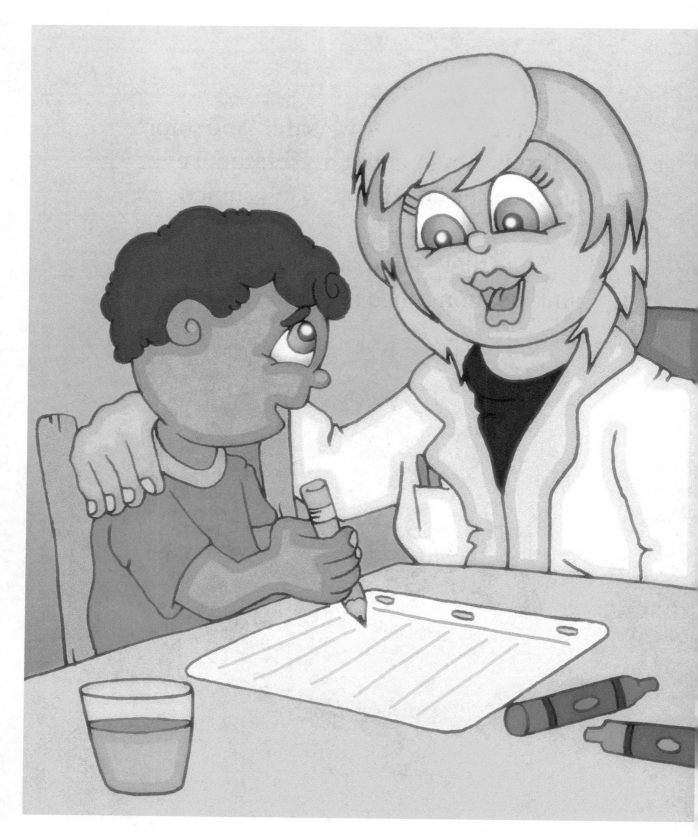

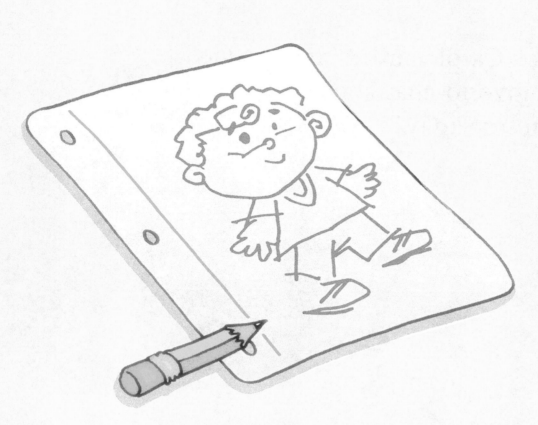

They talked about more ways Sam could help himself feel better after the awful thing happened.

On his last day of therapy, Sam said, "Ms. Carol, can I come and visit again some day? I'd like to talk more about my story."

Ms. Carol smiled and nodded, "I'd love to chat about your story again some day."

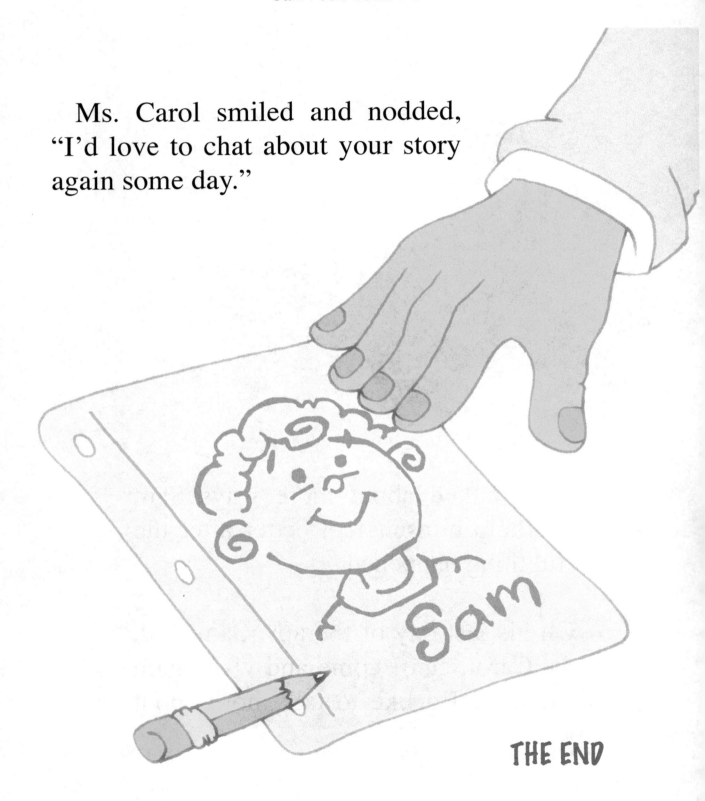

THE END

About the Author

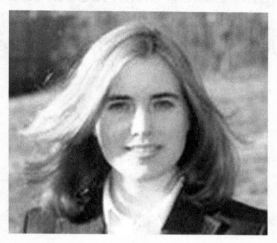

   Jill Osborne graduated from Toccoa Falls College in 2001 with a Bachelor of Science in Counseling Skills and Psychology. After that she went to work for the state of Georgia in a psychosocial rehabilitation and peer support program. During that time she went on to complete a Master of Science (M.S.) in professional counseling in 2006 and an Education Specialist (Ed.S) in professional counseling in 2007 from Georgia State University in Atlanta, GA. There she specialized in play therapy, traumatology, and child and adolescent therapy.

   During her graduate studies she interned and did contract work at Flint Circuit Council on Family Violence in McDonough, GA, for two years. Her experience there included counseling with women and children whom were survivors of domestic violence situations. She found her niche when she began using play therapy with children, and leading a support group for child survivors of domestic violence.

   "Sam Feels Better Now: An Interactive Story for Children" began as a project for a traumatology course taught by Dr. Greg and Dr. Cathy Brack at Georgia State University. It incorporates elements of trauma therapy, as well as play and expressive therapies to assist children in working through crisis situations, traumatic events, and grief by helping the character, Sam to feel better after his own difficult situation.

www.jillosborne.org

Therapist Guide
Therapist Guide and Resources from
"Sam Feels Better Now! :
An Interactive Story for Children"
Jill Osborne, Ed.S.

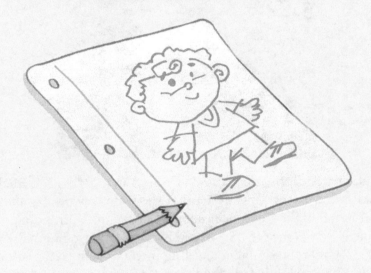

Sam Feels Better Now! : An Interactive Story for Children, (Osborne, 2008) integrates principles for trauma therapy, play therapy, and expressive techniques in order to assist the child through stage one of trauma therapy (Brack 2007). The story is appropriate to use with children ages 4-10 who have experienced a traumatic event, crisis situation, or are experiencing grief. It is recommended that children and parents who are interested in this story work with a therapist trained in child therapy. It incorporates expressive techniques and play therapy techniques, such as drawing, art, sand play, and storytelling to assist the child with learning various coping skills to decrease the effects of traumatic stress, anxiety, grief, and other symptoms he or she may experience. It is the goal of this book to create a fun, creative, and interactive experience for the child, and simultaneously provide therapeutic benefits by allowing the child means to relate Sam's experience to his or her own. In addition, it will assist the therapist in guiding the child throughout the therapy process.

The book can be divided into six general sections that address different aspects of trauma therapy for children; *Sam Meets Ms. Carol, Why Is Sam Scared, Sam Stays Safe; Sam Colors His Feelings, Sam Tells His Story*, and *Sam Says Goodbye* (Osborne 2008). Beginning in the initial stages of therapy, it includes relationship building, identifying potential symptoms, and normalizing of symptoms. After establishing a collaborative relationship with the client and parent, in *Sam Stays Safe*, Ms. Carol assists them in identifying a social support system. Then, they continue to create a safety plan for Sam. Further exploration of Sam Feels Better Now: An Interactive Story for Children, (Osborne 2008) promotes affect regulation, grounding, and stress management by identifying feelings, connecting body sensations with emotions, and utilizing relaxation techniques (Brack 2007) & (Briere 2006). Finally, at the end, in *Sam Tells His Story*, the child is asked to tell a story about Sam. This assists the child in preparing to tell about his or her own experience by using Sam's as a metaphor for his or her own (Kottman 2003). Following that is *Sam Says Goodbye*, which shows termination of the therapeutic relationship, and Ms. Carol leaving the door open for future sessions.

Many of the interactive components of the story are from Sam's point of view. This is done to create some distance for the child as they work through this book, in order to prepare them for telling their own story at the end of the book. Some children may want to directly relate it to their own experience. Therapists are encouraged to take the child's lead in this situation, and to encourage them to be creative throughout the child's experience.

Section headings are included in the Table of Contents as a guide for therapists who are using this resource with their clients. They are left out of the text of the story in order to create a seamless, smooth experience for children. A list of sections, their interactive components, and some suggestions is provided below.

Sections and Interactive Components:

Sam Meets Ms. Carol.

Can you draw a picture of someone who is scared?

Can you draw a picture of something awful or scary?

Why Is Sam Scared?

Therapist note: In this section, therapists may decide to work collaboratively with the children and caregivers to create a daily routine that is unique to each client.

Sam Stays Safe.

Can you draw a picture or make a collage of people that Sam can love and trust?

Can you draw a picture of a place where Sam can go in his house to feel safe?

Sam Colors His Feelings.

Can you help Sam color his feelings?

Can you help Sam by drawing ways that will help him to relax?

Can you help Sam by showing him where to color feelings in his body?

Sam Tells His Story.

Choose a way to help Sam tell his story. You can decide to use the sand box, puppets, art, or another Choose a way to help Sam tell his story. You can decide to use the sand box, puppets, art or another way.

   Therapist note: Allow the child to tell a story about Sam.

Can you tell a story about an awful, scary thing that happened? Draw a picture here, or choose another way to tell the story.

   Therapist note: Allow the child to make up a story of his or her own.

Sam says goodbye.

References

Brack, G. (2007, June 20). Stage 1: *Safety and security*. Presented at the 2007 meeting of the Georgia State University Traumatology Class, Atlanta, GA.

Briere, J & Scott C. (2006). *Principles of trauma therapy: A guide to symptoms, evaluation, and treatment.* Thousand Oaks, CA: Sage Books.

Kottman, T. (2003). *Partners in Play: An Adlerian approach to play therapy* (second edition). Alexandria, VA: American Counseling Association.

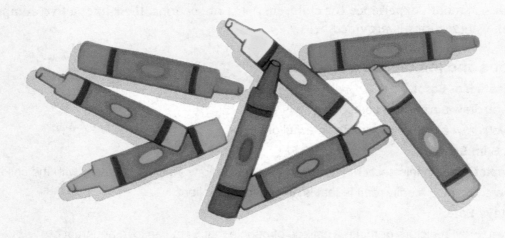

Resources

Books on Trauma:

   Briere, J & Scott C. (2006). *Principles of trauma therapy: A guide to symptoms, evaluation, and treatment.* Thousand Oaks, CA: Sage Books.

   Gil, E. (2006). *Helping abused and traumatized children: Integrating directive and non-directive approaches.* New York, NY: Guilford Press.

   Herman, M.D. (1997). *Trauma and recovery.* New York, NY: Basic Books.

Books on Play Therapy:

Landreth, G.L. (2002). *Play therapy: The art of the relationship* (second edition). New York, NY: Brunner-Routledge.

Kottman, T. (2003). *Partners in Play: An Adlerian approach to play therapy* (second edition). Alexandria, VA: American Counseling Association.

Books on Children's Artwork:

Cantlay, L. (1996). *Detecting child abuse: Recognizing children at risk through drawings.* Santa Barbara, CA: Holly Press.

Oster, G.D. & Crone, P.G. *Using drawings in assessment and therapy: A guide for mental health professionals* (second edition). New York, NY: Brunner Routledge.

Peterson, L.W. & Hardin, M.E. *Children in distress: A guide for screening children's art.* New York, NY: W.W. Norton & Company, Inc.

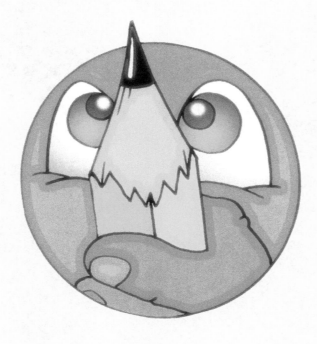

CPSIA information can be obtained
at www.ICGtesting.com
Printed in the USA
BVHW011125250620
582141BV00001B/30

9 781932 690606